DEDICATION

This book is dedicated to Emily Jane, our (Littlest Giant) who has fought for life even before she was born. To all children and other people with leukemia, I hope that this book will bring a smile to your face and brighten your day.

I want to thank all the students from Basha High School in Chandler, Arizona and the students from Northern AZ Academy in Taylor, Arizona for all their hard work to make this project a reality. Special thanks to Joe and Carol for helping out in such a big way with the family.

I appreciate St. Jude's Children Hospital for all that they do for children. St. Jude's ensures no child is ever turned away because of a family's inability to pay. St. Jude's is unlike any other Pediatric Treatment facility anywhere. Discoveries made here have completely changed how the world treats children with cancer and other catastrophic diseases. All who purchase this book, for 100% of the proceeds from this book will be donated to St. Jude's Research Hospital for Children.

My heart is filled with gratitude for the Marrow Foundation, the National Marrow Donor Program. To everyone everywhere that gets tested to see if they are a match for another to help save a life, I admire you!

Paulette Cleveland

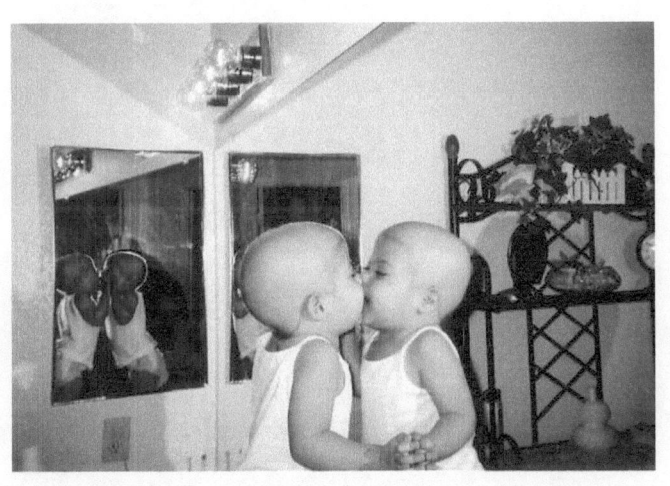

EMILY STILL NEEDS A DONOR

People everywhere donate blood to save lives, due to lack of knowledge about bone marrow and cord blood transplants many people never find a match. Give the gift of life for someone. Please help and get involved, get tested.

On any given day, more than 6,000 men, women and children are searching the National Marrow Donor Program (NMDP) Registry for a life-saving donor like you. These patients have leukemia, lymphoma and other life-threatening diseases that can be treated by a bone marrow or cord blood transplant. For many of these patients, a transplant may be the best and only hope of a cure.

We work to provide hope and deliver a cure to all patients in need. With your support, more patients can access the treatment they so desperately need.

For a successful transplant, the tissue type of a bone marrow donor or a cord blood unit needs to match the patient's as closely as possible. Special testing determines whether a patient and bone marrow donor or cord blood unit are a good match. The closer the match, the better for the patient.

Race and ethnicity matter in tissue matches

Because tissue types are inherited, patients are more likely to match someone from their own race or ethnicity. Adding more donors and cord blood units from diverse racial and ethnic backgrounds to the NMDP Registry increases the likelihood that all patients will find the match they need.

Your heritage can make all the difference. If you are from one of the following communities, you are urgently needed as a bone marrow donor or cord blood donor:

- Black and African American
- American Indian and Alaska Native
- Asian
- Native Hawaiian and other Pacific Islander
- Hispanic and Latino
- Multiple race

We have a Registry of millions. But we still do not have matched bone marrow donors or cord blood units for all patients, especially those from racially and ethnically diverse communities.

We need more new donors to join the Registry and expectant parents to donate cord blood. With your help, more people will receive a transplant. And more families will have a future filled with hope.

Join the bone marrow donor Registry and give hope to patients everywhere.

When you become a bone marrow donor, you join the global movement of more than 11 million donors who stand ready to give someone a future.

Even with millions available through the National Marrow Donor Program (NMDP) Registry, there are many patients waiting and hoping, unable to find a matching donor.

You could be the one a patient needs.

Contact Us

National Marrow Donor Program
3001 Broadway Street N.E.
Suite 100
Minneapolis, MN 55413-1753
The Marrow Foundation
3001 Broadway Street N.E.
Suite 100
Minneapolis, MN 55413-1753

- General information (NMDP or The Marrow Foundation):

- 1 (800) MARROW2 (1-800-627-7692)
- or submit a question <Sub-mit_a_Question/index.html> online
- The NMDP Office of Patient Advocacy: 1 (888) 999-6743
- or e-mail patientinfo@nmdp.org mailto:patientinfo@nmdp.org

CONTENTS

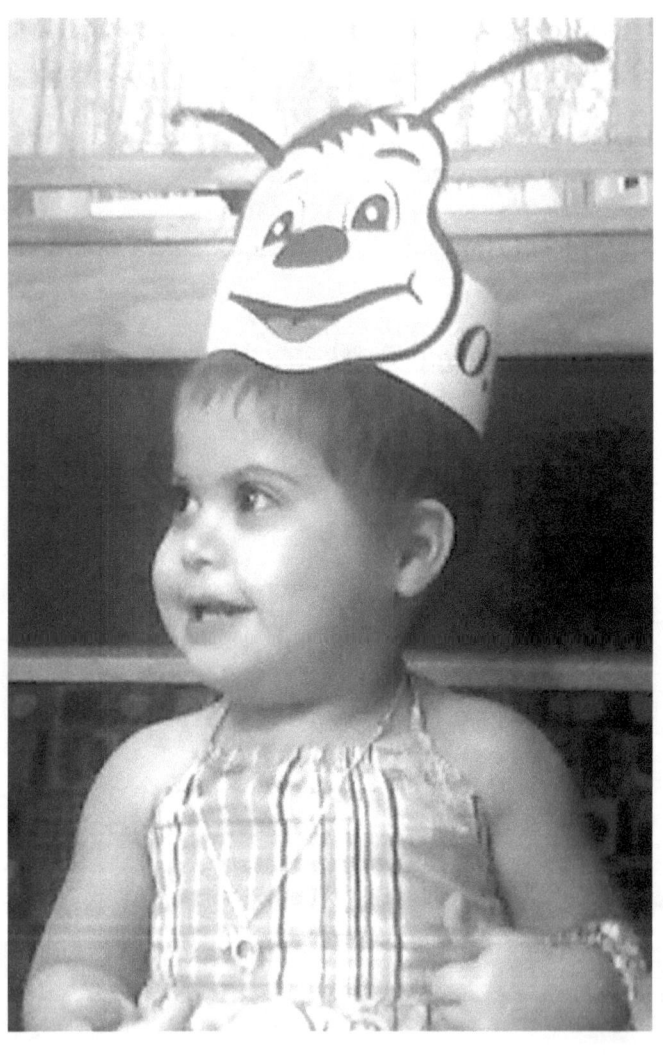

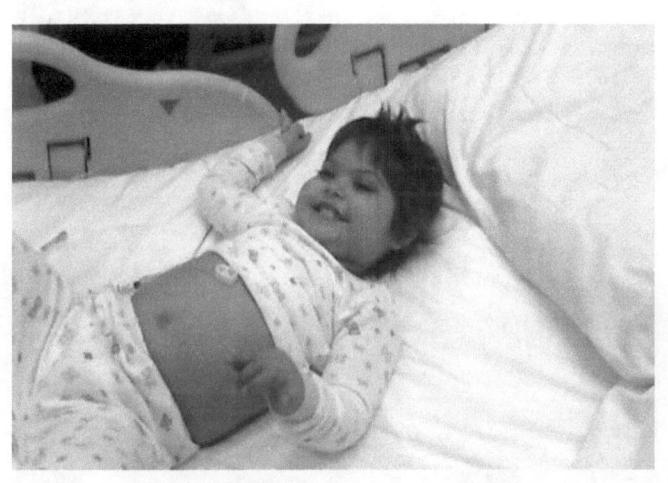

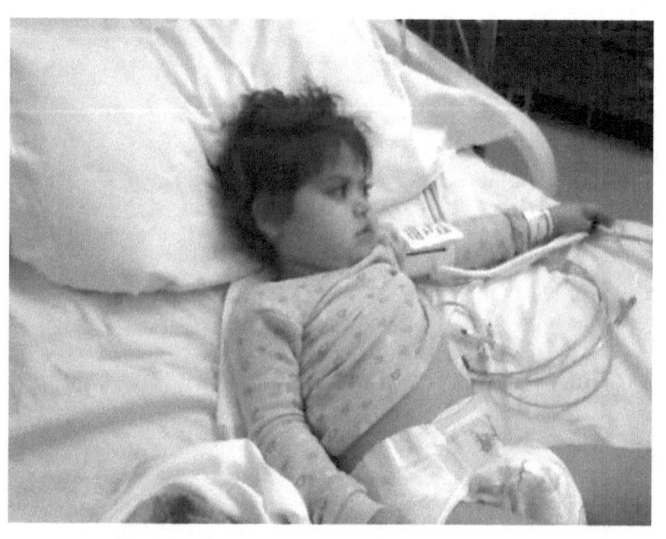

E...ncouraging

M...emorable

I.....mpressive

L....ove-able

Y....outhful

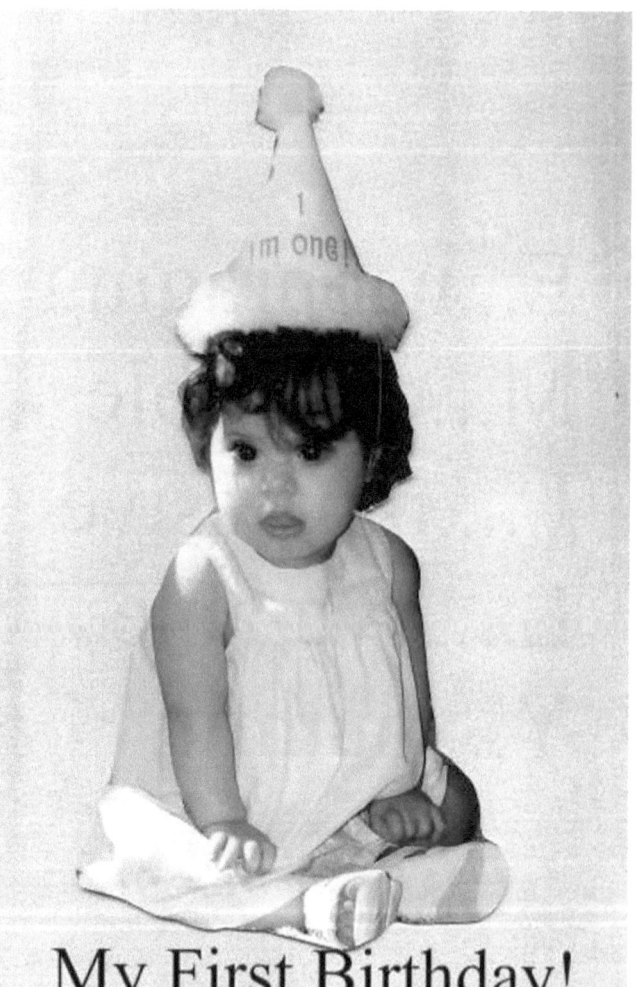

My First Birthday!

PRINCESS EMILY

Once there was a princess. Her name was Emily. She lived in a huge castle. One day she went to look around her castle. She went through the big door that took her outside. She's not able to go outside without her mom or dad. Then she went through the medium door that went to her parent's room. She can't go in there either. So she went through the small door. The door only she can fit through. There was an **awesome** playhouse with Pink walls and all kinds of "Build-A-Bears" all over the room with unlimited amounts of clothes.

THE END

Dawn Smith

EMILY'S SPECIAL DAY

It's early Saturday morning, I hear the pitter patter of little feet. Emily runs into wake Pop-pop. "Get up, get up, get up Pop-pop!" Emily says with a smile. Come on Pop-pop lets take a walk. Emily loves to go on walks with Pop-pop. Every day Pop-pop would take Emily for a walk outside. With her hair all a mess and her big brown eyes opened wide, Emily giggles as she jumps up and down on the bed.

Grandma Terry gives Emily a big kiss good morning. On the way to the kitchen, grandma puts on Emily's favorite music. Emily loves to sing and dance. Emily is very happy because today is a big day. It's Emily's special day! Today is the day that the doctor did say, that Emily can have cousins and friends come over to her house and play.

Mommy is busy, hurrying to get Emily dressed and all prettied up for her special day. "What color of dress do you want?" "The red or geen one?"

"And how should we fix your hair, put it up or in a braid?" "Come on now, hurry up! They are all on their way." Emily's mother did say.

The clock reads a quarter past two, the door bell rings and Emily screams with excitement and gleam! She runs to the door to open it, and who's waiting there? It's Jordyn and Julia with presents and balloons! With hugs and kisses they come inside. Into the playroom they run, pulling off their shoes and grabbing toys to share and play with.

Before you know it, there's a knock at the door. Guess who it is now? I bet you know. As the three them run to the door, it opens up before they can get there. In comes Steven, Brandon, Katie and Lauren each with a present for Emily. More hugs and kisses fill the room and everyone is happy. "Open your presents Em" says cup-cake Katie. Mommy says "You have to wait, their not all here just yet." And with a frown, they all sit down anxiously await the last two of the cousins to show up from out of town.

"It's hard to wait." says Julia, while Brandon puts his finger in the cake. Finally a car pulls up, and who do you think it is? Of course it's Evan and Ethan, they are the last two. They're here for Emily's special day. More presents all shapes and sizes, balloons of every color fill the room. Now Emily can open all her presents, eat cake and take pictures too.

What a wonderful day Emily had with all her

cousins and people she loves. A day filled with laughter, how sweet it has been! Now it's time for to go home. Emily says "good night" and mommy puts her to bed. Emily thinks about her special day, and with a big grin on her face, Emily falls fast asleep.

Auntie P.

THE LIFE OF A SNOWFLAKE

Life is like a snowflake falling to the ground. Just like us they all start out the same. All the snow-flakes come from high in the sky, all made if rain. Starting out their journey of life, a piece of ice that's hard and cold, falling to the ground. Not one snowflake is the same.

Snow is snow, but look closer now, millions and billions of snowflakes together make snow. Even though some snowflakes come from here and over there, higher and lower in a different parts of the sky. One way is their journey, down to the ground. Some snowflakes float down from the sky, while others come crashing down as the wind thrashes by.

Some snowflakes are quite large and crunchy and some are small and dry. Then there are those who are mushy and slushy, melting quite quickly and they seem to be very cold.

Like us, their life has a start and a end. Depending on the course they travel, they will be shaped and molded a certain way. As we experience life, we too will be shaped and molded much like the snowflake. We are so much alike and yet so very different at the same time.

Is one snowflake any better than another? They all come from the same place. They all fall to the ground and all have a beginning and an end. Some snowflakes last longer than others. Some snowflakes pile high on top of each other, while others just dust the greenery and the ground. Some snowflakes are eaten and others are thrown around.

Snow is snow its all the same, yet is so different too it's so hard to explain. Each with a different purpose in life and sometimes with no choice. So remember the life of a snowflake and make the most of your journey in life, cus we all start off the same and we will all have an end. It does not matter if your big or if your small. Speeding through life or just limping along. We are all so different, yet we are all just the same. The life of a snowflake is still a mystery to this day.

Margaret Ellis

"I JUST WANT TO SAY THANK YOU MOMMY"

I want to thank you mommy for loving and protecting me. I want to thank you for making me laugh and teaching me my A B C's. Thank you for all the times you made me whatever I wanted to eat, whether it was scrambled eggs or cheese and more cheese! It never mattered what time it was, day or night, you were always there for me. At times, I know it was incredibly hard to have patience with me when I could not sleep. Nothing felt right and nothing would do, up then down and up again, nothing felt right and nothing would do. No matter what, you tried to make it all better.

I want to thank you mommy for all those sleepless nights. Thank you for all the times you rocked me back and forth and softly patted my behind. You held me for hours on end till yours arms and hands went numb. I'm sorry for all the pain that you felt in your neck and back. Your body went beyond all that it could, because it was powered all by love. I am too young to tell you just where it hurts and what is wrong. Through my pain and discomfort you have always been there trying everything to help and make me all better.

I want to thank you mommy for taking such good care of me. For all the hospital trips and doctor appointments, there's too many to count. Only you could keep track of my crazy schedule and all those yucky medicines. Thank you mommy for being my rock and fortress of strength when everything seemed so bleak. I'm so blessed to have you for my mommy. I wish that I could tell you that I appreciate and love you. But seeing how I'm only three, you are just going to have to believe that my love for you is equal to the love you have for me!

EJS

HOPE

It had been a year since I last saw his face. One year exactly. It's hard for a fourteen year old girl to hear that her father was leaving for war. It wasn't something that I understood until it happened to me. The night he left is a night I can't forget; and the night he came home is one I will always remember.

It was at my fifteenth birthday party. I was so blessed to have my family and friends there to celebrate with me. I just couldn't keep my mind off my dad. Was he okay? Where was he now? Did he dream about me as much as I dreamed about him? No matter what, I never gave up hope.

I was so preoccupied cleaning up the wrapping from all my presents, I hardly heard the front door open. My mom called me into the room and I dragged myself out of the kitchen. He was standing in the doorway, covered from head to toe in his uniform. I didn't move. I didn't breathe. I took two faint steps toward him and let my tears build up. I

9

fell into my daddy's arms: finally. He cried and told me how much he missed me. I didn't speak. I just held onto him. There was nothing that could break us apart from each other. I have never held onto someone so tight before. I will never let go of my hero.

By: Angela Flores

WHAT I'VE ALWAYS WANTED TO SAY

You've always been there when I cried,
and always known when I've lied.
You're there to tell me good night,
and always know how to make things right.

You taught me how to read and sing,
and punished me when I did the wrong thing.
We may get in a petty little fight,
but we're always fine by the end of the night.

I look up to you Mom,
and I love you very much.
I don't know what it would be like,
without your loving touch.

I'll be off for college in less than two years
but I need to remind you as moving away nears,
you will always come first in my heart,

no matter how far we are apart.

I know I have not told you,
I don't know where I have been.
But you're not only my mother,
you are forever my best friend.

Tracy Reyes

MY CRAYONS

Today at school our teacher, Mrs. Rose told us to draw a picture of our family. I rushed to grab my box of crayons, some paper and I began to draw. Across the table from me sat Todd. He had blue eyes and red hair with lots of freckles on his face. Eager to draw my family, I snatch up a brown crayon, yellow then blue. I saw Todd grab the red, green and orange crayon. I felt very angry. How could Todd take my crayons? I took the white crayon and Todd grabbed the black crayon. Then there was one crayon left. The purple crayon. As we both eyed it, we dashed for it at the same time. Todd was much faster and got it before I did. Then Todd took the purple crayon and broke it in two! I could not believe my eyes and with my mouth opened wide, I let out a scream and started to cry. Mrs. Rose came over to see what was the matter. As she tried to comfort me, the bell rang and it was time to go home.

Later that day my mother came to pick me up

from school. She asked me what I did all day in school. I told her how Todd took my crayons and how he broke the last one. That night after dinner mother said "lets do your homework now." I got my backpack and reached in for my papers and guess what I found! My box of crayons all there and all fine. I felt bad for the way I had acted in school. Todd did not take my crayons. He even tried to share with me, breaking in half the last one so we both could draw.

Margaret Ellen

THE TINY RED LADYBUG

Once, in a very pretty garden, there lived a tiny red ladybug. For as long as she could remember, the ladybug had been very afraid of flying. She clung to the branches of the oak tree with all her might. Even when her family flew away for winter, the tiny red ladybug continued to hug her snow-covered branch.

"Why don't you let go, little one?" Asked a friendly robin, who was preparing to fly south. "The world is big and great and the skies are beautiful. There are roses to land on and sweet blossoms to smell. But if you continue to cling to this one branch you will never see such beauties, and you will never see your family again."

"I stay because I am scared", replied the tiny red ladybug. "This branch is all that I know, and it has been a safe home for me." "It is hard to fly with no one before you", agreed the robin. "But it can be done. You must be brave, and believe that no matter where you go, you will find love and compassion in the most unexpected of places."

The little ladybug stared at the robin with wide, innocent eyes. "I will try", she said, and she let go of the branch. And although her wings did not know how to fly, or where to carry her, the wind picked up the small insect and whisked her away, to lands of uncharted blessings.

Melanie Lammers

A NEW DRESS
FOR EMILY

It was a long ride in the car to the mall, but Emily didn't care. They passed the old white barn with lots of black and white cows in the field. Emily could see the mountain in the distance and she started to get excited, because that met that they were almost there, almost to the mall. Emily loved going to the mall. It was fun to go shopping. She liked to look at all the people and all the different stores, so many stores!

Today was especially exciting because Emily was going to get a new dress. She had been wanting one for quite some time. Because she had been a very good girl at home her grandma said she could go and get a new dress. Emily liked to get new dresses, they made her feel pretty. She thought about what kind of dress she might get. Maybe a big frilly red one, or maybe a baby blue satin dress with a big white bow!

Into her favorite store she ran and to her delight, dresses, dresses everywhere! They were here and there, high and low. From the front to the back of the store. There was big dresses and small dresses. Short dresses and long dresses. Purple, blue, green, yellow, orange and red. Every color of the rainbow. Black dresses, white dresses, even black and white dresses!

Emily didn't know which one to pick. She loved them all. Emily got sad for a moment cus, she knew she would have to choose one and just one. Which one will I pick thought Emily. I like them all, even those that do not fit! Emily looked for the prettiest dress, but she just could not decide which one it would be. Finally she turned to her grandma and told her to pick. Emily's grandma picked a multi colored dress, it was hiding in the back, stuck under all the other dresses where no one could see it. It had all the colors purple, blue, green, yellow, orange, and red. It had black buttons and a white bow in the center. It was long in the back and short in the front and it fit just right.

Emily was very happy with her new dress. She loved it and wanted to put it on right away! As Emily and her grandma were leaving the store, she thought, I have this beautiful new dress but I do not have any shoes that will go with it. Emily and her grandma went back to the mall to find some new shoes.

Olive Aria

FROG-GIE
"BABY TERRY"

The sky was bright blue and the sun was shinning over the hill as momma duck and her twelve baby ducklings swam in the pond by the corn field. Momma duck was teaching her babies how to swim and to be careful not to go out in the deep part of the pond. Big yellow daisys grew along the bank of the pond and a family of frogs live under a patch of beautiful red poppies. There was a Sally the mother frog, Fred the father frog, Harry, Barry and Terry, the kid frogs. Harry, Barry and Terry were all brothers. Harry was the oldest and the smartest.

On this day, Harry, Barry and Terry jumped in the pond and swam towards the ducklings. Harry told Barry, "I bet I can get there before you!" Barry said, "Oh yea?" By the time Terry, the baby frog heard what brothers Harry and Barry were talking about, both brothers were half way across the pond.

Baby Terry cried and he croaked because he was all alone. Sally the mother frog asked Terry, "What's wrong?" Baby Terry frog said "both Harry and Barry have swam across the pond without me." Mother frog told Baby Terry frog to dive in to the water, stretch his legs and swim very fast and far. She said "It will make you legs big and strong and one day you will swim farther and faster than your bothers Harry and Barry.

Baby Terry frog got very excited, he did as his mother said and jumped into the water, stretched out his legs and swam as fast and as hard as he could. When it was time to come up for air, Baby Terry was surprised to see just how far he had gone. His brothers were just a little bit away from him hiding in a clump of grass. Baby Terry dove down again in the pond, stretched out his legs and kicked and kicked as fast as he could. By the time he reached the clump of grass, Harry and Barry had jumped in the water and swam the other direction away from Baby Terry.

Baby Terry sat up on the grass and cried. Momma duck came over to see what was the matter. Baby Terry told Momma duck that his brothers were too fast for him and they would not wait for him or play with him. Momma duck told Baby Terry, "Well, this won't do at all." "You fall in line behind the twelfth duckling and I will teach you how to swim." "Oh would you?" asked Baby Terry.

"Come on now, Baby Terry get in line!" As

Baby Terry got behind the twelfth duckling, he swam on the top of the water. He could see all the little ducklings feet paddling back and forth as they glided across the pond. Baby Terry was happy to have so many new friends and to be swimming in a straight line. Because he was following momma duck and the twelve ducklings he could see where he was going and was able to cross the water much quicker.

Brother Harry and Barry had been swimming all day and catching flies on the lily pads. It was getting late in the afternoon when they noticed they hadn't seen their brother, Baby Terry. Being the oldest, brother Harry started to worry. He told Barry, "We better go find brother Baby Terry, before mother finds out he's missing." "Come on Barry, lets look over by the cherry tree and see if Baby Terry is over there."

Harry and Barry swam over to the cherry tree, but brother Baby Terry wasn't there. They went over to Dragonfly Island, but he wasn't there either. It was getting later and later and the sun would be going down soon. Harry new that his mother would be looking for the three of them to come home and eat dinner. Harry didn't want to tell his mother that they did not know where Baby Terry was.

Then around the corner came the momma duck. Harry and Barry cried, "Have you seen our brother Baby Terry?" Momma duck said, "Why isn't he with you?" Brother Harry put his head down in shame and said, "Barry and I took off this morning swimming fast and far away, Baby Terry is too slow to keep up with us." "It's almost dark and mother will be coming out soon." "Baby Terry is lost!" "Will you help us find him?"

Momma duck said, "look here, can you count how many ducklings I have?" Brother frogs, Harry and Barry started to count all her ducklings and when the came to the twelfth one, they saw a splash in the water. "Baby Terry!" "Where have you been?" "I've been learning how to swim far and fast!" "Meet all my new friends." Momma duck told Harry and Barry, "You should be nice to your brother Baby Terry, he might just save you one day!"

Harry and Barry were happy to have found their brother Baby Terry. The three of them swam home, all together and Harry and Barry were sure not to swim to fast for Baby Terry. That night at home, Baby Terry told his mother and father about his adventure in the pond. About all the friends he made and that momma duck was teaching him how to swim!

Later that summer, Baby Terry grew to be a very big frog. He was much bigger that his brothers Harry and Barry. Baby Terry grew right out of his name and was the fastest swimmer in all the pond.

PeeWee

MY FLOWER

"Come on Ashton!" A little eight year old girl called as she ran through the meadow. The boy simply scowled and watched her. "You're gonna get hurt," he warned. As if on cue, the girl fell, letting out a cry of surprise as she hit the ground. His eyes widened and he ran towards the girl, who was sprawled out on the grass, her coffee colored eyes looking up towards the light blue sky. She giggled as he frowned. "What were you thinking?" he scolded, "One of these days you're gonna to really get hurt!" She laughed.

"I don't have to worry about that, because you'll always be there to protect me." she said. She gave him a silly grin, in return he grimaced. "You know, you're the same age as me, and yet you treat me like a baby." the little girl whined. She stood up, mimicking Ashton's expression, and began looking around. Ashton merely sat down, frustrated at his friend, when he noticed something.

A lone flower.

It was pretty, yet at the same time, simple. The petals were and bright as the sun laid its rays upon it. To be honest, it reminded him of her. So fragile, yet pretty. So small, yet remarkable. He then turned around, and glanced quickly at the sun, which illuminated the white, delicate flower.

He smiled. He was the sun: giving her warmth, making her shine brightly... a big part of her life. She was the flower: relying on him. Needing him. He felt a hand tug lightly at his curly blonde hair. "Come on Ashton! Let's go to the park. I forgive you." The little girl gave him a tight hug from behind, and when she let go, he turned to her, and gave her a hug in return. The both stood up, and together, they both left the meadow. That day, Ashton vowed that he would always protect his flower.

Rianna Forcelli

HEAVENS GARDEN

Looking east I see the faint outline of the mountain top. Twinkling in the sky is the north star. The air is cool and crisp. In the distance I hear the chirping of the sparrows morning call. As I enter the north entrance of the garden wall a strong scent of orange blossoms surrounds me. The sun rays glisten like golden drops of honey on the dew covered grass. The sky is alive with beautiful pink, yellow and orange hues. I walk past the old white barn, where momma cat and her four black and white kittens cross my path. Happy to see me, she purrs and rubs up against my leg. The kittens chase each other through the hedges of mint and a wonderful aroma fills the air. A bright amber light shines through the windows of the barn giving a candle like effect in the background. I hear the sound of rushing water coming from the three tier fountain in front of me.

Turning to the right I go through a white picket fence, lined with English Lavender, Sweetpeas, Honeysuckle and Hollyhocks. Dense clumps of lavish flowers of woolly-silver, almost white; light blues, pinks, purples and reds stagger along the way. Music of wind chimes play their favorite song as a light breeze blows in my face and the warmth of the sun begins to cover the land. What beauty feels my eyes. A glorious feeling over comes me as I see my grandmother sitting on a bench across the field. She sees me and motions for me to come near. I love her smile. Her eyes are so bright and blue. Running to her is so effortless. With so much emotion, my heart feels like its going to explode. As I finally reach her, she bends down to hug me. I hold on to her with all of my might.

Suddenly in the back ground a noise emerges. It starts out faint and begins to grow. Louder and louder it becomes. I am disturbed by this unpleasant and unwelcomed sound. I can not identify it and it won't go away. Why won't it stop? Make it stop, please make it stop. The strong smell of black coffee now fills the air. I open my eyes and see the sunlight shinning in the window. I reach over, turn off the alarm and get out of bed. On my way to the kitchen I pass grandma's picture on the hall wall. Remembering my dream, I smile and think of Heavens Garden. What a wonderful place. The memory of my grandma would put a smile on anyone's face. Walking through Heavens Garden fills the heart, soul and mind with all the pleasures one could bare, oh what a great and happy way to start each and everyday!

Paulette Cleveland

NATURE

Nature is the endless sky,
The sun of golden light,
A cloud that floats fairly by,
The silver moon of night.

Nature is a sandy dune,
A tall and stately tree,
The waters of a clear lagoon,
The great waves on the sea.

Nature is a gentle rain,
And winds that howl and blow,
A thunderstorm, a hurricane,
A silent field of snow.

Nature is a peaceful breeze,
And pebbles on a shore,
Nature is each and one of these,
And infinitely more.

Written by
Daniel Armando Munoz
10-10-81 -- 12/20/07

***

This poem was written in 1994
and won the 6th grade <u>Earth Day </u>contest
at Sierra Middle School Tucson, AZ

UNTITLED

Life for Ali was great. She had it all. She had the loving family, the cute shoes that all the other third graders wanted, and most of all the best friend. Her best friend's name was Samantha and without her, Ali was nothing. The two were exactly alike and did everything together. Their fellow classmates envied the true bond Ali and Samantha had together. Everything seemed wonderful and glorious when one day Ali called up Samantha and told her that she needed to tell her something very important and that she needed to come by right away.

Samantha quickly ran downstairs, told her mom she was going to Ali's, and grabbed her bike to ride to her house. Samantha got there and Ali was waiting at the door for her. Ali sat Samantha down and told her that her beloved dog Frootloop died. Ali was devastated and cried in Samantha's arms for hours. Samantha, being the great friend that she was, told her that everything was going to be alright and that she was there for her no matter what. The two friends got through that tragic day and many others that followed in on going years.

Ali and Samantha were friends much longer after the third grade. They grew up together and grew old together. Even though their lives sometimes went in different directions, the two always seemed to be there for one another. A friendship that is inseparable should forever be cherished as Ali and Samantha cherished theirs.

Keshet Miller

LEILA'S
GOODBYE BEAR

It was early in the morning on a cold and windy
November day, when Leila was being discharged
from the hospital. She had been in the hospital again
for more chemo. As Leila and her parents walked
down the long white corridors of the hospital, she
noticed that they were coming up on room 245.
Leila broke free from her mothers hand and started
to run. When she got to the door it was closed. She
tried to open it but could not. This was the room
that Emily was in. She had only known Emily for a
short time. She wanted so badly to say good bye
and give Emily the picture that she had drawn for
her. Emily's grandmother went to the door and was
surprised to see Leila. Leila's tiny body and little
bald head tried to squeeze by. Emily, Emily cried
Leila. Emily's grandmother said " I'm sorry Leila;
Emily can't have any visitors today". Leila's big
brown eyes filled up with tears. Leila said, "but I'm

going home today and I want to give this picture to Emily." Leila's mother pulled her away and said "Come on honey, you know that Emily needs her rest."

Emily's grandmother saw the hurt in Leila's face and said "Oh Leila, I'm so sorry that you can not see Emmy. I will give her your beautiful picture. I know she will love it." Leila and her parents went back to her room to wait for the doctor. Emily's grandmother put the picture next to Emily's bed, because Emily was asleep. She went down to the gift shop and found the prettiest bear she had ever seen. It was big, fluffy and pink. The bear had great big white angel wings on it. Emily's grandma bought the angel bear, took it to Leila's room and said "this is from Emily. She wanted to say good bye and thank you for being such a good friend." "This is a Good bye Bear and it has big beautiful white angel wings so he can watch over you when you go home." Leila grabbed the bear and kissed it. It was love at first sight. Emily's grandmother looked up at Leila's mother and they both had tears in their eyes. Leila's mother said "Leila, say thank you." Leila ran to Emily's grandmother, giving her a big hug, and said "Thank you!" The doctor came in the room and told Leila that she could now go home.

Katlyn Anne

DAY AT THE RIVER

Along a river bank, two fairies flew just above the water. They chased each other left to right, up and down. They chased each other till the fairy in the lead came to a halt. "Hey, Mathis, lets make it fly," said the first fairy pointing at a frog with one hand and pushing her purple hair out of her face with the other.

"No, Isabella, remember what happened to Casey?" called Mathis. She was not as fast as us," taunted Isabella, as she edged closer and closer. "Isabella!!! called Mathis, "You're going to get hurt!!!!!" Isabella, however, stuck out her tongue and flew closer and closer. With one croak and a splash, the frog leapt into the river. Isabella was drenched from head to toe, as Mathis burst into laughter. "I told you so," called Mathis as he laughed harder and harder.

Isabella, however, splashed Mathis so Mathis splashed back. For the rest of the day, they splashed each other and played. Never play with things that can hurt you.

Nicole Laws

MEETING BIG·DADDY

"Hi, I'm Danielle!" I said shyly, extending my small hand to the tall man standing in front of me.

I was meeting my Big-Daddy for the first time ever, and he looked taller than tall... especially to a five year-old. He put out his big hand, and in the biggest voice I had EVER heard, said "Hi, Danielle, I'm Harry, but you can call me Big-Daddy!"

I turned to look for my sister who was staring boldly at him. "Hi, I'm Casey," she said. Then, with a tone that was less than friendly, stated "You're really tall!" (My Mom gave Casey a tiny swat on the behind.) "What"?! Casey responded, her bottom lip sticking out, her arms defiantly crossed in front of her.

Big-Daddy's voice boomed as he laughed out loud and his whole 6'5" frame shook. "It's okay", he said. I was staring at him and thinking "Wow, I wonder if i'll ever get that tall !!!!!!"

He looked down at me and said to my Mom, "I just can't get over how much like you she is, especially from when you were young." I looked up at her and she nodded, smoothing back my hair. I shook my head and it went right back to normal.

Big-Daddy just smiled...and, like every other part of him, that smile was BIG. We left for burgers......knowing that we had the BEST GRANDPA ever!

Danielle Cairns

AMBER AND ANDREA

My two little girls,
One's like a big mommy
While the other was kind-of scrawny

Blonde hair with blue eyes
One loud and one shy

One's tall and the other short
So much alike,
But so different you see...
One looks like her daddy
and the other one, like me

Oh what a blessing
That God has sent me two
Nothing could be better
Because he sent you

Now that time
has passed me by
You're much bigger

And so wise

I'm so glad I am your mother
could you imagine any other?
You would not be who you are
And I could not reach for
My favorite star

All the years together,
I would never change
No, not now
Not ever!

I love my girls
And will always be
A very, very
Special part of me.

Love, Mom

A BUTTERFLY WING

"Time is a wild thing," my Mama used to say. "You've got to watch it like a hawk, and grab it quick when it tries to slip away." She'd slide behind me where I lay on her tattered hammock, rocking it so violently that I squealed in mock-terror, her giggle making me grin.

She'd make herself comfortable with my young body in her lap, taking my wrists into her worked-chapped hands, and stretching them out so we reached to Time together. "And hold on tight now, honey, it's slippery as a snake, and moving faster than a horse can run." We grabbed at the stars, clung to the moon, and stretched out our groping fingers for Time. "You don't want to let go now, honey," she'd whisper, "caused once you lose Time, there's no getting it back."

Her voice crooned in my ear, the familiar words comforting and warm as the night closed around us. The hammock swung us back and forth on a breeze,

Mama's body cradling mine until we both fell asleep under the sky.

I never knew how precious these moments were until Mama was gone, and Time finally made her loose the firm grip she had on its slippery hide. That's what she was trying to tell me all along; Time is a priceless, one-time gift--irreplaceable.

A butterfly wing tickles my ear:
"That's right, honey--treasure Time--it's the only way you can ever really hold on tight."

Taylor A. Collins

YOU WILL BE
REMEMBERED

*To: Patty Ann Walker, Grandmother, mother, wife
& friend.*

Some will be remembered for the fortunes of their fame, and some will be remembered for the naming of a name.

But you will be remembered as the heart remembers spring, as the mind remembers beauty, and the soul each lovely thing.

You have been skies of April, and fragrant breath of May. Like the seasons coming, warm, spirited, and gay.

You have given freely of the beauty of your heart. You have made of friendship not a gesture but an art. You have been as selfless in the gracious things you do as the sun that shared it's kisses and the night that shares it's dew.

You have planted many roses in lives that lay so bare. And you have sown encouragement to those who only knew despair.

By spirit's inner beauty and in every lovely thing. This is how I'll always remember you.

As the heart remembers Spring.

Vicki Lee Wakefield

MY GREATEST
VALUE OF LIFE

My family gives me joy, strength, and support
My Family gives me my morals to carry throughout my life
My Family gives me unconditional love
My Family gives me happiness, hope and love

My Family gives me promises and plans for a future
My Family gives me understanding in troubled times
My Family gives me trust and respect of who I am
My Family gives me a listening ear and a hand to hold
when needed

My Family give me lasting traditions to continue in
my life
My Family gives me freedom to make choices in my life
My Family gives me guidance
My Family gives me celebration and hope to a bright future

My Family gives me appreciation for who I am
My Family gives me privileges

My Family gives me inspiration to dedicating my life
to others
My Family gives me wonderful memories to fill my heart
forever I will always have my, Family

Mandi Craghead

DREAMS YET TO BECOME REALITY

In Loving Memory of Edith Winograd
&
Sherry Ann Dern

Ever since I was a little girl I have known that one day I want to become a doctor. Not until four years ago did I know what I wanted to specialize in.

Four years ago, my great-grandmother, Edith known as GiGi, passed away from oral cancer and old age. Just two and a half years later, my grandmother, Sherry Ann, passed away from having breast cancer for twelve years without remission. Both of these women were amazingly strong, always had good attitudes, and smiles on their faces. I admire these women for their courage to keep fighting and their knowledge of how to make every moment count, that of which they passed on to me.

One day I want to prevent others from the pain they endured by becoming an oncologist. I am more that willing to go through the extra schooling.

My dream has always been to somehow make a difference in the world, even if it's small. I am aware that the career I'm pursuing will have many highs and lows, but for me the highs will be extremely rewarding. To know that I could save just one person's life and spare their family the pain of loss would make every bit of it worthwhile. This will be the dream that I make a reality.

Becca Dern

E IS FOR EVAN AND E IS FOR ETHAN

These are my two grand children, boys from the start. Evan is the oldest with a lot of heart. Ethan came into this world at the beginning of summer all bloomed out like a giant flower. Evan chose to enter into life as the weather started to cool. He has colors of whites, blues and purples like when the snowflakes fall. Ethan busted through the warm earth growing and twisting while reaching for the sun.

Evan is like taking a walk in the park and seeing a nice white park bench and sitting there for awhile. Taking in all the sights and sounds learning from his every turn. Being quiet and listening to mommy and then practicing over and over until he's going to win.

Ethan is like running through the park. He's excited to see what's ahead. His short legs and broad shoulders make him waddle in the sand. He watches the other kids, but still he has his own way. He's got to be more daring, or maybe it's the best way. Up the ladder way up high then with his big ole belly on the slide, head first he comes and then arrives.

Over and over again, he can't get enough. And what is this crunchy soft stuff beneath my shoes? I'm not quite sure but when I put it in my hands it falls apart. Tiny rocks and they stick to my hands. I rub them together and watch the fall to the ground. I bend over and grab two more fist full. I like the way it feels and then just disappears.

Big brother Evan, he knows how to count. Forwards and backwards. The alphabet is nothing for him to spit out, mix up all his flash cards and he can point them out. Evan loves to play his Mario Brothers game, he hops and jumps along with the characters and can even blow flames out of his mouth with his buddy Bowser. Then its time for WII another video type game. From boxing, fishing, playing a game of pool, identifying and picking out Danny, Nicholas, Angel, Ethan, Daddy, Mommy, Grandma, Antie, Windy, Nick and Gammie in a dark room, running or swimming by you can pick them out incredible fast and you've got the best time! Even racing cows is not hard for you, sometimes just for kicks you run those cows into the fence.

Such a big boy and your getting so tall now. Learning to read, add and subtract- you're like a big leap frog because you listen well. You started very early even before you could actually walk. I wonder what you will become someday. Will it be a doctor, a lawyer maybe a school teacher or cop. Maybe you'll become a football star or a great golfer and teach daddy a thing or two. What ever you choose, it will be done with care and precision with a gentle touch.

Little brother Ethan isn't quite so little. He is thicker and wider. I call him my little football player! I think there should be "Toddler Sports" for the little ones who just can't sit still. Always on the move, can't slow down and exploring every bend. Food is to eat and eat he does do, then he finishes up what his big brother did not do. You can see in his face so much love and happiness. His eyes light up and he's happy to see you. He's got this walk, it's really very cute, he sort of waddles side to side when he runs around the house. It almost looks like he just got off from ridding a bronch.

Ethan is here, there and everywhere. He's happy go lucky, not a sissy boy at all. It's up for a hug and a kiss- then let me down! I have much to explore, so get out of my way! I wonder what Ethan will be someday. Seems like a wrestler, since he practices every day. He'll probably be in sports 'cus you can't hold him down! But then his inquisitive side shows up quite clear as he tries to figure things out. He walks around the house with this puzzled look on his face with his eyebrows scrunched up to one side, such a serious look as he runs by I wonder what he is in?

Ethan is the type that doesn't want to be left behind,

he will sit with his big brother at the table and try to write his words and letters. And he will do his best even when Evan and mommy sing. But in no time at all he's off like a flash, where to- don't know but he'll find out when he gets there. Even getting out of the bath he has no time to be dried off with a towel, he might be missing out on something in the other room. Running out of reach he dries with every step, just a few seconds until momma comes, what can I do that I know I should not?

Ethan is growing fast and soon will be much bigger than his brother. It will do, for right now to run up and side swipe Evan off the couch and wrestle him to the ground. Evan gets annoyed, because he's playing WII. Eventually, because they are brothers, they both wrestle and fall to the ground. Laughing and kicking and seeing who's the strongest. At the moment Evan has the upper hand, but not for to long. Evan will have to out-wit Ethan because by the looks of it Ethan's going to be what I call my "BIG OLE COUNTRY FRIED CHICKEN EATTING MACHINE." Right now I call him Tank!

I love my grandsons, Evan and Ethan they are so different, just like **(night and day)** and just like my daughters Amber and Andrea **(cold and hot)** Our genes are such a wonderful thing. Now I am waiting for by blond hair blue eye little girl from Amber to balance things out. We can't let the boys have all the fun! I can just see it now, the little princess with all kinds of attitude to keep those boys in line all the time. No pressure here Amber, take your time. But for now I love my grandsons, Poppeye and Bubba, what a wonderful life for me.

Love, Grandma

DANCING

Once upon a time there lived a young girl in the middle of the forest; it was just her mother, her father and her. Many people would visit the small family just to watch the girl dance. "One, two, three! One, two three!" said the little girl as she danced her dance.

One night a man came to the small family's home. "I'll give you a hundred dollars if you dance for me," the man said to the little girl. So she began to dance. "One, two, three!" said the little girl as she danced once more.

"Very nice," said the man getting to his feet as the little girl finished. With a smile he said, "Now, I will give you two hundred dollars if you never dance." "Never dance again?" asked the girl with a quick glance at her mother and father. Then she said to the man, "Dancing is my life and I love it. Never in a million years will these feet stop dancing." With a smile she danced again, and the young girl danced for the rest of her life.

Nicole Laws

UNTITLED

When the news came that my grandma had cancer, I didn't know what to think. The fact that she might die just didn't really sink in. I felt numb inside. I never thought it could happen to my family. She went in for chemotherapy, and my mom called her a lot. I knew she was really lonely there with all her family away. As the weeks went by, nothing really changed. I asked mom how grandma was doing to make her feel better and offer my comfort. She was going through a really rough time. Mom was depressed a lot and Grandma had no one to talk to. She would cry at night and have no shoulder to lean on. I wondered why there was no one there for her. Then the news came. My grandma had survived the cancer and was free to go. Everyone was really happy that she gets to live and dance and enjoy life for another year. We are going overseas for their eightieth birthday this winter. We're staying for Christmas too, and the whole family will get to be together. Then everyone will be able to support each other. I was shocked that something that seemed so distant could hurt my family, but it turned out alright in the end. I just can't wait to see her smiling face again. -Auzrill

Alix Haugen

MY SISTER

On October 7, 1993 my mother had fought for
the last three months
of her pregnancy to keep her second child, my
brother's twin, alive.
She had done all she could
and now came the day
for two lives to be brought into this world.

When my brother came out successfully
everyone rejoiced and
to this day we still do, but then
my little sister came and her
little lungs could not breathe.
She was too fragile
and too delicate
to be able to withstand this heavy world.

God made her my guardian angel
and I believe she lives on through me.
Some days I look at my brother
and imagining what she'd be like

and this poem
lets the whole world know
that I have not forgotten her.
Despite the fact we only rejoice on this same day
every year for my brother,
I do the same for my sister.
I love her
and believe
she's always been here
to guide me and
always will.

Rebecca Suarez

A LIFETIME'S NOT TOO LONG...

I have moved seven times. I know to many, seven is a small number, but the story is just the same. Five of the seven moves have forced me to leave friends behind and make new ones at a fresh placed called home.

Every time I've moved, I've thought, "Why now? After making such great friends I have to leave?" These questions have lingered in my head the past few times I have moved, each move having them linger a little bit longer and becoming more dominant in my thoughts. Every time, I wonder, if people were meant to have friends, then why are we made to leave them? Or, if people move so much, why have friends at all? But consider this, when you move have the people you left behind truly left your heart? Have they left your thoughts forever? Just because you don't see them anymore, doesn't mean that ther're not your friends anymore.

In my last move, a particular song helped me remember the true meaning of the phrase 'BFF'. The lyrics go

"But we'll keep you close as always It won't even
seem you've gone
'Cause our hearts in big and small ways
Will keep that love that keeps us strong
And friends are friends forever
'Cause the welcome will not end
Though it's hard to let you go
In the Father's hands we know
That a lifetime's not too long to live as friends."

"Friends" Written by Michael W. Smith and Deborah D. Smith; Produced by Mark Hammond; Performed by Jump5

Branden Waller

AMANDA

I could've gone with him. When he packed his things, left his apartment and emptied what was left of his ravaged bank account, I could've done the same. When he set his sites for Washington, D.C. I could've joined him. I could've brushed the dust of that little town off myself and gotten out. But I didn't. Instead, I stayed behind. For Amanda.

Several years ago, on a warm, sticky summer afternoon Amanda called me. I didn't know her, but that didn't stop her from rattling off an address in my ear and telling me she expected me for lunch the following afternoon.

A slave to my undying curiosity, I went, and to my surprise arrived at the gates of the local nursing home. Amanda seemed out of place at first. She was a striking woman, as vivacious then as she'd been at twenty-five. When I questioned her, she told me that slowly, she was going away. She told me that was why she'd wanted me to come; so that she'd still be able to look back, even if she couldn't on her own.

Her memory was failing. While Amanda could remember the dress her mother had worn to her wedding, she stumbled with the name of her newest grandchild. It hurt me as much as her own children to see her struggle, but I dutifully wrote every word.

Then Amanda went away. I remember that day. I stood over Amanda's grave with her eldest daughter, and I remember wanting to leave as well. To leave the town that held all the places she'd told me about. So when he asked me to go with him to Washington, I was ready. Carefully I packed my things, but I couldn't leave. I realized why. Amanda hadn't recounted her memories for herself. Amanda had recounted them for me.

When I started this story, Amanda was a young girl, much like Emily. But as it grew and developed, Amanda did as well, maturing from a small child struggling with illness to an aged woman trying to hold onto her past. Amanda came to resemble my mother's late grandmother, Leona Knos Hansen, who died in 1995, at the age of 88. A sweet and caring lady, Grandma Lee developed a severe case of Alzheimer's Disease towards the end of her life, which escalated to the point where she couldn't remember my grandfather's name before she passed away. She told my mother stories about her life, which my mother passed down to me, along with a ring my great-grandmother left to me in her will. I tell this story in her memory.

Ana Domovoi

WHITE DOVE

Spending my last moments
with the family that I love,
when laughing and playing together
I saw a beautiful, White Dove.

I thought for a moment
as it glided through the sky,
that maybe after all,
it wouldn't be bad to die.

While we were laughing and playing,
I lay down on the ground,
when all of a sudden,
it was blue and clear around.

I looked down on my family,
where they wept and cried,
before I came to realize
that sadly, I had died.

I know that they'd be happy

now that I was above,
watching over everyone
just like a beautiful, White Dove.

Michelle C. Harrington

MY SISTER

For someone I never knew
My heart aches when I remember

The pits of regret that lie in my heart
Are for her name that is never spoken and I constantly forget

She would have been my friend I think
I'd have her while my brother and sister had themselves

I cry sometimes when the day is near
Wishing I could have just seen her face and remembered

Just imagining her grace and beauty
Never-ending

She would have smiled a lot like me
Happiness

My brother would be changed
Difference

Life in her sole instead of in heaven
Beautiful

Rebecca Suarez

***

I wish I knew her today
Everyday we'd sit and play
Live, laugh and learn to see
The world around us and what it'd be

She'd be my sister and my friend
Loving each other until the end
I wish God would have given her a chance
To live life, be free, and dance

Her memory is sadly vague
But I love her anyway
When I reach heaven, if I do
I'll greet her gladly with arms open...soon

Rebecca Suarez

FAMILY

Stuff seems so scatter

Like stars in the sky

But it all comes together

And I feel so alive

I know they are

They let me know they are there

Even though they are far

Every time they sing

It almost makes me cry

I can hear the bell ring

In the back of my memory

I love them so much

As they have loved me

I'm glad that are here and there

They are my wonderful family.

Monica Viesca

OVER·FILLING ECHOS

Gracious
Polite
Cordial
Courteous
Attentive
Approachable
Kind
Friendly
Neighborly
Thoughtful
*
Grumpy
Unkind
Inhospitable
Sharp
Rude
Unsociable
Disagreeable

TJ Brown

UNTITLED

The seasons are changing and leaves are flying.

It feels like all your love is beginning then dying.

Looking up at him wishing I could undo it all.

Then opening my eyes and seeing tears fall.

I have to sew my heart strings back into one,

before they all come back undone.

Believe believe is all in my mind.

And the speaker sound is beginning to wind.

Up the streets down the waterfall.

I love the way you show it all.

I will follow you like you follow your heart.

Please don't let me fall apart.

I see angels in your eyes.

Not even they could give the disguise.

Jacqueline Shelton

WHY

I thought you would always be there
Never thought you would leave
You always seemed concerned about my feelings
Asked about how I was doing

One day I tried to ask you about a question but
you didn't answer you were to much in
A hurry you packed your things and
Walked out the door, though in my heart
I knew you were lying, I started crying

I didn't understand
Did you do something wrong
How could you leave for so long
Mom wouldn't eat,
I couldn't sleep
Friends were asking questions,

And before long, faint memory
Back then, we needed you
I would wait by the door thinking you would

Come home but then I grew up
And learned to live without you

Now looking back, I see how much you missed
All the pain you put us through
I realized, it wasn't my fault
I was able to move on and stop living in the past.

Carlye Nino

LOVED ONE...

I'm so lost
In this world with out you.

It's cold
And all I see is darkness.

As I walk down the street,
As I clean my room,
As I fall asleep,
All I see is you.

My head is blurred,
And all my thoughts stop in their tracks.
They know I need you.

You were my best friend,
The one I could talk to.
You were my family.
I need you,

But I left.

I didn't want to leave,
But I left.

I see your smiling face,
On snow white walls,
I miss you.

You were my favorite,
But I left.
I'll come back,
To live with you one day.

Oh dear Nelson
You were my family,
And I need you.
Now do you understand?

Amanda LaCasse

"VIEW"

I saw you sitting on a bench.
In your hand was a wrench.
We humans never realize
What is up in other lives.

I saw you laying on a bed.
Bandage wrapped 'round your head.
We humans never realize
What goes on in other lives.

We can't seem to find the time
To give the needy their last dime.
Our ignorance won't realize
What goes wrong with other lives.

These are words I do dread.
Go back home to tombs instead.
We humans just can't realize
What's up in other lives.

David Moss

WHY, OH WHY

Why, oh why,
Must you suffer,
The way you do.

Why oh why,
Must you have,
This disease.
It consumes you,
It eats you,
What can you do.

Why, oh why
How old were you,
Nine,
Five,
Or four,
When you got
This awful curse.

Why, oh why,
This curse,

This disease.
Did it choose,
A child
Like you.

Why, oh why
Does it pick
On little kids,
And older ones
As well.

Leslie Kay Tobara

THE BATTLES OF CANCER

Lying here tonight;
Scared to know if I'll wake up right.
Wondering if I'll lose my hair;
Though some wouldn't care.
Sad to look in the mirror and see;
The reflection of little me.

What will others think?
Stares that make me want to shrink.
Can't they see its only me?
But no, they won't let it be.

Its okay, I won't mind;
Beauty inside me I will find.
One day in heaven they will see;
The beautiful, confident little me.

Sarah Klein

YOU

I love you,
Forever and always,
I do,
No matter what happens,
No matter what,
I do,
Or say,
I love you,
More and more,
everyday.

Leslie Tobara

SOFT·CUTS

Forgive
Disregard
Excuse
Exonerate
Ignore
Absolve
***
Revenge
Detest
Avenge
Hate
Dislike
Resent

TJ Brown

IN THIS REFUGE

In this refuge,
I can't see you.
In this silent room,
You're here.

I need to stop this blindness,
To reopen my eyes.
To see again,
To feel, to touch again,
These voices
Comforting till after
The effects.

Cursing, blaming runs us.
The rest follow hard after others
Followers of lesser people,
Slain to the rest,
Dead to our conscious,
We live no more inside,

Why we live is forever going

Unanswered.
One answer, no question.
We need to die
To live again, being
Firm is too hard for us,
And being weak is our strong
Point.
For others to follow,
After lesser people.

Looking in the mirror
Nothing shows
But something else
Reveals all.
Not wholeheartedly seeking,
Partly even standing
To be near him,
We turn again, to
Follow after lesser
People.

TRUE LOVE

You are my superman always there with a plan

When I fall you grab my hand you are always there for me

To care for me and to share with me you swoop

Me up when I am down and catch me before I hit the ground

The light in your eyes could brighten the skies in which

You Fell from you are and angel from above

Your eyes are why we fell in love sent on the wings

Of a snow-white dove I have given you my entire heart

From the beginning, from the start I have

Nothing left to give yet you love as if I did.

Shelly Sharp

SOMEONE LIKE YOU

Someone special,
Someone cool,
Someone like you,
Forever,
Someone weird,
Someone right,
Someone like you,
Forever,
Forever.

Leslie Tobara

LOVE

There are many words left unsaid

Many repeat over in my head

The way you look at me each day and say what's in
you heart

Makes me think, maybe I'm not so alone when
we're apart

A soft touch

A starlit sky

A perfect night

With you near by

Your beating heart is a melody that never lies

With eyes of castles and blue skies

In the lonely days of sorrow and fear

I think of when you were near

I'll be here fighting

For you forever,

And ever on

My love will remain strong.

Jody Arredondo

YOU ARE SPECIAL

You are special,
Not like anyone,
That I know,
You are my,
Best Friend Forever,
Don't you know,
You understand,
My feelings,
Better than
Anyone else,
You are special,
In every way,
You are,
You are awesome,
You are perfect,
You understand,
Everything I say,
You are special,
In every way,

You are you,
In every way,
You are.

Leslie Tobara

LIVE

Laugh like no one's laughing

Sing like no one's listening

Dance like no one's watching

Dream like your dreams will come true

Live today like it's your last

Love like you've never been hurt.

Janine Vanlandingham

SPECIAL

I was in an accident,
My scars still hurt,
How no one seemed to care,
Except him,
His name is a secret,
That I keep in my heart,
No one can know,
What he meant,
To me,
How much he understood,
He was to me,
The best friend,
That it is possible to have,
He treated me,
Like a daughter,
Him like the father,
That had never,
Been there.

Leslie Tobara

THIS OR THAT

Beauty
Attractiveness
Cuteness
Fairness
Gorgeousness
Handsomeness
Loveliness
Prettiness
Allure
Attractiveness
Glamour
Elegance
Exquisiteness
Flawless
Radiance
Desirable

*

Unattractiveness
Foulness

Homeliness
Ugliness
Dreadfulness
Ghastliness
Flaw
Grotesqueness
Hideousness
Offensiveness

TJ Brown

INDEFINITE LOVE

Love is a feeling I cannot explain
I feel happy, perfect and complete
Love is a feeling that can't go away
It is something that I'll always need
It defines who I am and who I'll always be
I think about it everyday
Love never fades, no matter what happens
I love her in every way
I'll be hers forever what ever happens
I love her in every way
I'll be hers forever what ever it takes
I always want her in my life
Someday I hope she says yes to me,
When I ask her to be my wife
She is amazing and I am not
I don't care what anyone thinks
She is the love of my life, my everything
Being away from her makes my heart sink
She's my one and only and she always will be
I hope she feels the way I do
We've stuck together for better and for worse

And I know love is what got us through
I know I'm not perfect and I've made some mistakes
But love has changed me it's true
No matter what happens I hope that you know
I will always love you.

Jordan Smock

MARTIN

Thick family history
surrounded by mystery

Fresh air and purple mountains
With blue skies
The waves rolling in
With no lies

Times of good
Times of the past
Our time together
Will always last

Laughing or
Crying
You always are smiling

Up and down
Good and bad
Oh, what things
We've never had

Miles and miles
of the beach we did walk
Knowing each others
voice-less talk

Endure, endure!
Until the very end,
Oh what a wonderful friend
That you've been

I'll meet you there
someday, somehow
But until then
Remember me- remember me

I will always pray for you
And know that my love is true
Now, with a kiss
I wish you only
peace and happiness.

PM Cleveland

YOU CAN NOT UNDERSTAND ME

You cannot understand,
How I feel!
You cannot understand,
How I see,
The world around me!
You cannot understand,
Anything about me,
Unless,
You go through,
What I go through,
Everyday of my life,
Unless you do,
Then don't
Ever,
Say that you understand,
'Cause you don't,
I promise.

Leslie Tobara

A WISH

Is there a possibility
For happiness, for me,
Sometimes I wish someone,
Would hold me,
Tell me of all that
They feel for me,
Make me feel loved,
And safe,
Make everything
I've done okay.
Eyes locked,
On one another,
My one true love,
To be there no matter what,
To console me,
Be with me,
Hug me,
A part of me,
To see the real me,
Not be criticizing,
Take me as me,
Not something fake.

Even if I change my ways.
It's just a wish,
Though,
Never to change,
Always,
Except
For my baby boy.

Antasia Gillies

NOW AND THEN

Lively
Energy
Spirited
Bouncing
Animated
Frisky
Gay
Vivacious

****

Lazy
Sleepy
Criticize
Weary
Dull
Boring
Lifeless

TJ Brown

MY LIFE IS
IN YOUR HANDS

My life is in your hands,
You're in charge,
Of What happens next,
So don't make me cry,
Don't make me hurt,
Hold my life sacred,
As your own,
'Cause,
My life is in your hands
You keep me alive,
Or make me die,
My life is in your hands.

Leslie Tobara

UNTITLED

I will make something of myself
Despite what all might say
I won't arrive
At the gates inscribed,
"Abandon all hope upon entrance here,
For only pain and suffering are near."
I will not fall with all the no-names and die,
Who threw away their empty lives
I will stand up and make my say
So the world will know my place
I will bring forth change
And leave my name
In the hearts of men
And rumors unsaid
I will make something of myself
Starting today
And the world will never be the same.

John Ralston

THE LIGHT DARKNESS

Love
Care
Enjoy
Respect
Delight
Appreciate
Cherish
Treasure
Adore

****

Despise
Neglect
Abandon
Hate
Depreciate
Detest
Dispise

TJ Brown

MY FRIEND,
CAROL SHELTON

Carol, Carol Oh what a gal,
Who could forget that southern bell?

What beauty was inside
As you learned to abide,

Finally discovered and brought to life
Sacrifices were made,
While you paid the price.

Carol, I miss you
and am glad you were my friend.
Angels above the
Lord did send.

The lives that you touched
And the friends that you made,
You are leading all heaven now

In a glorious parade!

***

***In memory of
Carolyn Ann Shelton
1953-2007***

Paulette Cleveland

CRY

If you never cry,
How do you know,
How it feels,
To lose someone,
That you love,
Unconditionally,
If you never love,
You can't know
What this feeling,
Feels like.

Leslie Tobara

WANTED TO

I wanted to know what was taken
I always look low what was mistaken
Desire is such a game
In such of an age
Being wasted to the tastiest smiles
Being on there side I felt so satisfied
Friend is a cherished one
Whose proven task can be done
Nights are always in my sight
Always fun under the moonless light
Maybe dark but still can smile bright
Sleep is the only thing we had to fight
Might think my mind is corrupt
But I never past misjudgment
Happy among myself
I always would be felt.

Chaira

HOW

Life is so difficult,
It is hard to see,
The person,
That you should be,
A person that,
Through it all,
Has always been there,
For everybody,
You have been
Through some hard times,
Where you have wanted
To protect everyone,
You love,
Your family,
Your friends.

Leslie Tobara

"UNTITLED POEM"

Sixteen years of age
So young
So innocent
So full of life
Now gone.

Taken,
Snatched,
Painfully ripped away,
Snuffed out, without a care,
A bright angelic light, extinguished before m eyes,
    as tears stream down my face,
Now gone.

Music surrounded him,
Notes, rhythms, melodies danced through the mo-
    ments of his life.
The fun,
Love,
Excitement,
Rush of life, so full of opportunity,
Now gone.

Stolen from this world,
So young,
Innocent,
Full of life,
To leave behind
Family and
Friends.

The world seems a little less bright as each year passes.
One,
Two,
Three,

His smile,
His laugh,
His happiness,
Now gone.

Gone on to a better place, where he may smile,
Laugh,
And love,
For
Eternity.

-Danielle Campanella

BEAUTY

Beauty is here,
Beauty is there,
Beauty is simple,
Beauty is pleasant,
Beauty is inside and out,
Beauty is YOU!!

Leslie Tobara

A DAY

A day is what you make it,
It can be fun,
Or it can be bleak and boring,
It can be wonderful and exciting,
Or it can be dark and sad,
A day is what you make it,
So make it what you want.

Leslie Tobara

HELL FROM
THE OUTSIDE

Don't you know why I didn't
Help you out?
Point you in the right direction
And help you seek another way out.
From inside you hurt,
And from the outside you bluntly
Acted it out,
Your whole life a betrayal
Of what you really felt.

You know your feelings, I didn't
But discernment is a gift.
I saw you, felt you anger and frustration,
You've been alone for a while now
But why I didn't help...
Don't know why.
So many chances,
Even just one would be enough,
To make your life different,

Less tough.

Just once, I would like to do it
All over. To redo and try again,
If I could I would give you my
All,
You would see a difference
In me and my actions
Decisions, words, and specially you.
Don't know why I didn't
Help you out.
But that's gonna change
Today, right now
No more sittin' and bein' selfish
It's over,
I have to help,
Otherwise
You'll see Hell from the Inside.

Becoming leaders, we fall
But get up only to follow
After lesser people
But we live to die,
For him and
Our eternal soul.

Josiah Huggins

UP AND DOWNS

Everyone goes through those up and downs
Every once in awhile.
I have to admit that I go through them all the time.
It is hard for me to go through them.

I need my closest friends always by my side to
Get me through them. The one that
Knows everything little about me
I am grateful that I have those type of friends.

Most of my up and downs are with my friends.
When we look back on what had happen we realize
That wasn't a huge thing that we made it out of.
I can get mad at them but the we work it out
We get through it.

Some of my up and downs come from boys too.
Especially the ones that you actually like of think
Is cute.

I wish there were up and downs in my life.
Without them my life would be a whole lot better.

Candice Kennedy

SILENT EXPLOSIONS

Peaceful
Calm
Tranquil
Submissive
Quiet
Yielding
Mild
Serene
***
Hostile
Fierce
Combative
Aggressive
Forceful
Billerengent

C.C

THE WORLDS
SOUNDTRACK

Artistic passion;
Flowing rhythms
Match a strong beat,
Creating beautiful melodies
A painted picture
Illustrated by words the lyrical outline
It complements the song
G,C2,E-
Float to the ceiling
A story told by music
About tragedy, achievement, and love
One mans secrets;
The world's soundtrack.

Bransen Caperton

ALWAYS ENDING

Praise
Blessed
Celebrate
Extol
Glorify
Magnify
Laud
***

Rebuke
Blame
Criticize
Admonish
Reprimand
Lambast
Censure

TJ Brown

HOT RED

I am speed, I am speed
Rev my engine, feel the need turn my key and
Hear me roar let me loose, petal to the floor take me
On the highway and I can soar fuel injection lets me
ascend
Even more like a blade I pierce through the air
Other cars snicker and snare five point seats, glossy
paint
So smooth and sleek street racin' at midnight
My owner says its "so tight" touch my hood, you
might get
Burned watch me glide into this turn I'm a 65 Ford
Mustang running free through the valley my owner
Says she can't live with out me thousands of explo-
sions going
On under my hood open me up, I think you should
22" black walls on the street feel my motor rumber
under
Your feet Kenwood speakers make me stylish take
Me to the car show and I'm the wildest cost two
grand

To step inside this grab my wheel and feel the rush I
Turn asphalt into mush see my signature in
The Street just glance at you and me can see the
heat
I under go the wrench in the garage
When you see me finish you'd think I
Was a mirage.

Shelly Sharp

WHAT IS LEUKEMIA?

Leukemia : acute lymphoblastic leukemia (all) . It is the most common form of childhood cancer. It affects lymphocytes, a type of white blood cells. Leukemic cells accumulate in the bone marrow, replace normal blood cells and spread to other organs including liver, spleen, lymph nodes, central nervous system, kidneys and gonads. In the united states, about 3,000 children a year are found to have acute lymphoblastic leukemia. Peak incidence occurs from 3 to 5 years of age. About 98 to 99 percent of children with newly diagnosed acute lymphoblastic leukemia attain initial complete remissions in four to six weeks. About 80 percent of children can be cured. Patients who remain leukemia-free for 10 years or more can be considered cured. Chemotherapy is used to kill leukemia cells. All chemotherapy is stopped after two to three years of treatment.